POSTURE BOOK

Gabriela Condrea

Bodhisattva Janet,
I hope that the little
reminders within these pages
inspire you to feel just a little more
rooted and hold your crown just a
little higher. We each have the
power to inspire those around us —
on the dance floor, in life — because
good posture is contagious.
un abrazo,
Gabriela

PAINT WITH WORDS PRESS

Seattle, Washington

DISCLAIMER:
This book is intended for educational and informative purposes only and is not meant to diagnose or treat a medical condition or serve as medical advice. If an injury or other condition makes these exercises painful or otherwise uncomfortable, or if any of these movements cause pain or discomfort, discontinue and consult your physician or other healthcare professional about your unique needs.

CONTENTS

Introduction   pg. 5

I. Imagine   pg. 9

II. Head to Toe   pg. 25

III. It's All Connected   pg. 77

IV. The Base, The Source   pg. 89

V. Down & Up   pg. 101

VI. Expand   pg. 119

VII. Let's Take a Walk   pg. 131

VIII. Awareness   pg. 151

IX. Self-Connection   pg. 175

INTRODUCTION

A little book to help you feel a little taller and a little more in control of your posture and your space.

Since 2010, I've been helping people connect. A lot of this work has to do with posture, because how we carry ourselves impacts our balance, our confidence, our health, and the way we interact with the world around us. And my students joke that they're getting taller! Of course, we can't add inches, but we can choose how we use each inch of height we do have.

Tips for how to use this book:

Posture is a practice you cultivate. It's about building awareness and good habits – and to build new habits and create new neural pathways for ourselves, repetition is key. With this in mind, this book is full of little reminders, imagery and cues to help build new posture patterns, to help you build a daily posture practice.

A little bit at a time… Throughout this book, you'll find images and concepts all with the same goal: to help you align your posture for a more comfortable, more efficient you. Choose one or two to work on at a time – for a few days, a week. When you feel you have incorporated it solidly into your body, come back for another image or concept. Perhaps you'll be inspired to come up with your own imagery or visualization (I'd love to hear about it on our social media). It's not quantity, it's quality and being able to discern what works for you – now and as you progress and your needs change.

Build in "pit stops", like a race car driver, cues for yourself to check in with your posture. When I see this, I do that. Every time you hit "send" on an email, for example, or when the timer on your watch or phone goes off, during each pause in a song if you're a musician, or build in a pause here and there if you're dancing, as I tell my students. Perhaps it's every time I get up to go to the bathroom, I stretch my arms above my head. Since I'm not there to give you cues (unless you come to my classes), find cues that work for you, preferably naturally-occurring ones that happen throughout your day as reminders or "pit stops" to check your posture.

Empowered. In life, there are many things outside of our control, our sphere of influence. How we carry ourselves is a small, yet profoundly consequential thing we can in fact influence. Of course, an injury or medical condition might create challenges. Even so, take a look at my TangoStride™ students and how empowered they are, even in the face of tremendous obstacles. There is so much we can choose for ourselves, and that's what this book is about.

Finally, there is no precise, proper way to stand. We are all structured a little differently. The imagery and references herein refer to physical ways of holding ourselves – not to individual peoples' structures or shapes. Meet yourself where you're at and explore what feels good in your body. You are your best advocate. Keep what feels good and leave the rest. When you revisit this work in a month or two, perhaps you'll find other tidbits that feel good to you. It is your journey – own it and savor each and every moment.

IMAGINE

Posture is a dance

It's not like you "get" perfect posture and then hold onto it. Posture is fluid and shifting, adapting and changing. And we have choices at every point in this subtle dance, in each moment. What posture is best for how you are moving right now, for you to move and be the most optimal version of yourself? What about now? And now?

Wear your crown

Imagine you have a crown[1] on your head. Don't lose it! Don't let it fall off the front of your head, the back of your head, off one side or the other.

---

[1] Inspired by Mariana Dragone.

A daisy flower

Stretch toward the sun.
Stretch your stem long,
leaves out wide.
Reach your crown
unapologetically
toward the light,
soaking in
every
ray.

Chin up, Buttercup. Keep your head up.

Posture is internal

We see it on the outside, but what we see is just an outward expression of what's happening on the inside – like the outer rings of the ripple when you toss a stone into water. We are the center of that ripple and what we do within us is expressed on the outside... and ripples on out in space and time.

Balloon guy

Car dealerships often have them, stores, fairs, big balloon guys flopping and waving and dancing in the wind. Every once in a while, they fill up with air and expand, big and tall and wide. Then they flop again. This is a fun warm-up for our classes, but you might do a "balloon guy" during a break at work, to start your day, or whenever or wherever you need a little flopping and expanding action.

I like to pair this with music to inspire me. Put on a song and let it guide your movements. I imagine the music is my wind, blowing my balloon self around, and every once in a while, the music tells me it's time to fill in my balloon and stretch big and wide.

Pineapple

I saw a meme about standing like a pineapple and it just tickled[2] me so! I was smiling to myself the whole day, saying "Be like a pineapple. Stand tall and wear a crown" – had to tell all my students. It's perfect for our image of the crown – regal, poised. Plus, pineapples are so sweet and tart, they make me think of sunshine. The image made me smile. Perhaps it'll make you smile, too? Stand like a pineapple.

---

[2] "I'm just tickled" as my friend Nikki would say.

El junco y el roble

"Although an oak tree (el roble) is stronger than a reed (el junco), the reed can better withstand the powerful winds of a storm – instead of fighting the wind, it sways with it."[3] We need to be strong enough to stand tall and bear weight, yet elastic and flexible enough to be able to adapt to changing terrain and circumstances, to shift and move with ease.

---

[3] Gabriela Condrea, *When 1+1=1,* (Seattle: Paint with Words Press, 2011), 19.

Puppet on a string

Imagine there's a string holding you up through your center, coming out of the top of your head, like a puppet. You just go bouncing around, lightweight and carefree, underneath this string. You don't have to hold yourself up because this imaginary puppeteer with his imaginary puppet string does the work for you. Perhaps there are strings to lift your arms, too.

Stacking

We are designed to be stacked: feet, hips, shoulders, head. Where are your hips in relation to your feet? Where are your shoulders in relation to your hips? Your head in relation to your hips and shoulders and feet? If someone were to look at you from the side, would they see your head centered over your shoulders, hips, and feet?

Imagine a Jenga® tower of blocks or a stacked rock statue. If stacked just right, they stand upright without any extra help. How can we use our positioning and alignment to make standing, balance and posture feel more effortless?

Head over heart, heart over pelvis.[4]

---

[4] A common yoga cue.

Good posture is contagious

Have you noticed how when someone straightens up near you, you feel the urge to check your posture, too? Even just at the mention of anything about posture, people often adjust their body almost automatically.

By adjusting your posture, you might inspire others. Improve your posture and you might just start something.

Good posture is contagious!

Friends don't let friends slouch

"I wouldn't let you slouch," said Ron in class one day, "and you wouldn't let me slouch."

I thought about it.

"You're right, Ron," I answered, "friends don't let friends slouch."

Like a dancing flame,
a swaying tree,
a blade of grass,
– dance.

HEAD TO TOE

Posture is a full-body sport

Crown

A reminder to check your crown. In our classes, we just say "crown" and the students and I check the position of our heads and our crowns. One of my students, Joni, actually brought a crown to class one day. My student Steve takes his hands and puts on an imaginary crown. He'll remind me, "I have my crown on my head." And of course that means I need to check mine, too. Thank you for the reminder, Steve!

Where is your crown? It could be helpful to look at your reflection in a mirror the first few times you adjust your crown to have visual feedback to pair with the sensation: How does it feel in my body when my crown is straightened?

Check. Your. Crown.

Head floats

My student Ellie told me that her yoga teacher would say, "head floats, shoulders down, elbows back" and we'd repeat this many times in class. It takes time and reminders to build a new habit and the muscles to support it.

Ears up

"Lift your ears up," my yoga teacher Lucy Greene would say, in her 70s with impeccable posture. Where are your ears? Could they be lifted more toward the ceiling or the sky? Imagine some little hooks on strings or cranes gently lifting your ears…

Eyes eye level

"Eyes on the horizon," tango teacher Susana Miller says in her classes. Look out at the horizon as far as the eye can see. What happens to your head?

What if you had laser beams shooting straight out from your eyes? Where would they be pointing? What would they burn a hole through?

Where our eyes go, so does our head. Keep your eyes eye level.

Eyes on the prize

What is your "prize"? Keep it out in front of you so you know where you're going, what you're striving for – and make it tall. Keep your eyes on the prize. I had a student who I would say this to. He would lift his head a bit, yet his gaze was still angled downward. I'd say, "Make your prize a little taller." He'd laugh and lift his gaze some more.

Relax your face

My Bunica "Granny" Raia would tap her forehead to remind me to relax the creases in my furrowed brow. Do you feel tension in your forehead? How about your jaw? Are there muscles in your face that are working even when they don't need to be? Do you feel a correlation between a tight jaw or furrowed brow and tightness in the neck, upper back, and chest muscles? Can you squeeze your muscles tight as if you just took a bite of a lemon? What about wide like surprise? Shock? Awe? Joy? Delight?[5]

---

[5] Inspired by Candy Conino's game of facial expressions and the yoga cue to relax the muscles of the face.

Where is your chin?

Where is your chin? Is it sticking out in front catching snowflakes? Is it tucked away hiding from the sun? What is a neutral position for your chin?

Turtle shell

Is your neck hiding in a turtle shell? Come on out…

Be gentle and patient with yourself, especially if the turtle has been hiding for quite some time. But do make your way out – we need you out here!

Wrinkles out of your neck

Is the back of your skull sinking down toward your upper back? Is your neck compressed?

"Take the wrinkles out of your neck," says instructor Adriene Mishler on the at-home yoga video I'm following along with. This just automatically makes me lengthen the back of my neck.

If when you lengthen your neck your head is pulling forward on it, see if you can stack it more over your shoulders, spine, pelvis, center.

Make your neck long.

Are you looking down to look up?

Some of us look down by bending at the lower vertebrae of our neck so much – while reading, writing, typing, looking at a screen located lower than eye level, looking at our feet – that we forget to straighten up before looking up. When we want to look up, we just lift our eyes by bending at the upper vertebrae of our neck creating an S-shape, like a vulture.

Rather than keeping the bend in the lower part of the neck, let's straighten it out first. Start from the lower neck vertebrae and unfold, lengthening upward. Now that the neck is in a neutral position, adjust the head from the place where it sits on top of the neck. The head goes up to look up, down to look down, from the upper vertebrae of the neck first. If we need more range of motion, then add the other vertebrae in. For example, if looking straight up toward the ceiling, you'll likely want to start the movement lower in your neck, even your upper back if it is a really big movement. We want everything working in concert.

"Are you looking down to look up?" Candy Conino asked us in her anatomy class.

Texting while looking down?

So many people are looking down at little screens while sitting or walking.

How about lifting your phone to you rather than curving your upper back and neck toward the phone? Feels like more work, doesn't it? But when you put your head forward, your upper back and neck muscles are stretched and have to work hard to hold your head from falling forward. That's hard work, too.

A touch of the upper back

In tango class, when my students come dancing by and they're a little collapsed or hunched in the upper back and neck, I gently touch their upper back. They know this nonverbal cue and straighten up, stretching tall through their upper spine – and the rest of their body.

Shoulder shrug

Have your shoulders crept up to your ears? It can happen gradually, almost sneaking up on us… before you know it, you're up to your ears in shoulders! Let's exaggerate this with a shoulder shrug. As you inhale, pull your shoulders up toward your ears even more, as high as you can, then exhale and release, letting them drop. You can do this once or several times in a row. Repeat as needed, every time you catch your shoulders creeping up to your ears…

Sometimes it helps to exaggerate the movement to emphasize how silly it is that the muscles are working so hard. When your muscles feel how overworked they are, it can help them remember what it's like to relax. They'll be like, "I deserve a vacation!"

Shoulder slide... ahhh...

Many of us hold tension in our shoulders. We worry about this – shoulders go up, we worry about that – shoulders go even higher. We want to reach something, hold something, pick something up – shoulders ride up, up, up. All this work for our upper back and our shoulders. It can be hard to undo all at once. So, perhaps start by developing awareness. Where are my shoulders? What are they up to? And let's create this little habit: every time you notice your shoulders creeping their way up, breathe in, breathe out and release. Just say, "Thank you shoulders, I got this." Ahhhhh…. And let them slide on down your back.

Notice, breathe and release.

Balance in the back

Are your upper back muscles and shoulders too enthusiastic?[6] Are they doing more than their fair share? Let's recruit those middle back muscles into the party. Gently pull your shoulder blades downward and inward toward midline using those muscles just between and below your shoulder blades, the rhomboids and lower trapezius. Get them to give your upper trapezius a break!

---

[6] Inspired by Lonn's "enthusiastic" pepper.

Shoulder shimmy

We often think of shoulders moving up and down, perhaps forward and back, but they also twist. "Walk" your shoulders forward, one at a time; walk them backward, one at a time... You can even lean a little forward as you shimmy forward and lean a little backward as you shimmy backward. If you're sitting, slide your hands forward and backward along your thighs as you go.

"C" shape vs. seal shape

An agile spine is a healthy spine. Our muscles get used to a position and shorten or lengthen in accordance. They respond to our use of them. Make a rounded, curved-in "C" shape, bringing your chest toward your pelvis, moving your belly button and the middle of your spine backward. Then alternate this with arching your spine the other way, bringing your belly button and middle back forward, your upper back and butt closer together in the shape of a seal holding itself up on its front flippers, extending, sunning its chest and face.

Maintaining range of motion is vital to a free-flowing, moving body – and it gives you more options when it comes to your posture, too.

Are your shoulders closing in on you?

Some people move about the world with their shoulders sort of closing in on them. How are your shoulders positioned? Are they rolled inward and forward? Are they perhaps rolled out and backward?

Let's open and close the chest and shoulders. Bring your shoulders forward and in and then out and back, closing off your heart space and then opening your heart space. You can add in your arms, too. Do this back and forth until you settle on somewhere in the middle, a comfortable in-between neutral position. Moving to the extremes is a great way to keep yourself flexible. We can't just hold a "happy medium" all the time. We are meant to move, breathe, flow. Movement is life.

Unzipper your heart

Rori Raye says, Imagine you have a zipper in the middle of your chest. Unzip it. Unzipper your heart.

Lighthouse

Imagine you are a lighthouse emanating life-saving light from your sternum.[7] You have the light ships need to see. Don't keep all that good stuff to yourself – shine it far and wide!

---

[7] Inspired by an exercise Rodolfo Dinzel used to do with his tango students.

Be around your spine

Imagine a column or rod going through the very middle of you. Your body rotates around it when you walk, when you dance. Anything you do, ask yourself, Where am I in relation to this column? Where am I in relation to my spinal column?

Move using this as the center, the core, the origin, the place from which you generate movement. Twist around your column, notice how it stretches and bends. We spend so much time and energy "in front of" it; *be* around your spine.

Let your ribs "drape" from your spine

Let your ribs "drape" from your spine, versus you having to "hold" them up there – or "hang onto" them, says Feldenkrais practitioner Ed Mills. Trust that they are attached and they're not going anywhere.

Move yo' ribs!

"Did you say 'ribs'?!" my student Gus says, "I like ribs!"

Our ribs are meant to shift and move, expand and get farther from one another, contract and come closer together. Sitting or standing, how can you move to shift your ribs farther apart on one side of your body, then the other? On the front of you, then the back of you? Can you breathe in a way that moves different parts of your ribs? How about a little dance with your ribs?

When your ribs get "stuck", it can impact your body all the way down to how you position weight in your feet, says Ed Mills. When our ribs move freely, our whole body moves better.

Have you met latissimus dorsi?

You can hold your posture with your latissimus dorsi ("lats" for short). How? one might ask. The lats are the biggest muscles in the upper body, and they pull on the bottom corners of your scapulas (shoulder blades). This is how they can indirectly affect the position of your shoulders, chest, neck, and head.

Hold my scarf with my lats? Wait a minute, how can the lats on the back of my body "hold" anything? Well, it is in fact true that the lats cannot grab hold of something. However, by positioning our shoulders in a way that feels more aligned, it can feel so much easier to carry something. That's why I had the sensation that when I engaged my lats to pull the corners of my shoulder blades down, the scarf in my hand felt almost weightless.

Dance with your back

When we talk posture, a lot of focus is on the front of us. Much of our life happens "in front of us". We especially focus on the chest and shoulders (even in this book, I had a lot to say about them). Yet we have large muscles in our back, and far too many latissimus dorsi and the oft-forgotten lower trapezius are going under-utilized. Do a little dance with your back, especially the middle of your back. Now how do your shoulders feel?

Back back

Where in relation to the rest of you do you tend to hold your back? Are you leaning forward? This could be at your middle back, lower back, or even your pelvis, hinging at the hips. It could even have to do with where in your feet you're putting your weight and with your ankle mobility. What if you brought your back backward, in line with your feet and hips? "Back back," I tell my students.

Wings

Imagine you have wings coming out of your shoulder blades. Where are they? Are they sagging to your sides? Engage the muscles in the middle of your back, pulling the scapulas down and into the center, repositioning and preparing the spots where your wings would attach.

I had a student who would lean forward and downward a lot, afraid of falling. Perhaps this gave him the illusion of being safer. Yet it made it hard to keep his balance and made a lot of work for the muscles along the back side of his body. "Use your wings," I would tell him and reach my hands behind his shoulder blades, gently drawing in the air his imaginary wings up and back so he'd straighten his posture.

We did this with my student Nancy, too. She even started showing off her wing, extending her arm proudly out to the side.

Bowl[8]

Imagine your ribs are a bowl facing upward. This bowl is filled with a liquid. If you ask my student Gus, he'd tell you there's some special TangoStride sauce in there that he made himself. What's in your bowl? As you move about, careful not to spill it on yourself. Imagine a dance partner in front of you – you don't want to spill it on them either. Not to one side or the other. Walk or sit keeping the rib cage "bowl" level so as to keep all that special sauce from spilling.

---

[8] Inspired by Alicia Pons' "bowl" exercise.

Like putting on a jacket[9]

Some of us walk around with our ribs sort of splayed out. Let's bring it in, team. Engage the upper abdominal muscles, just enough to support you. Imagine hugging your ribs toward each other and inward toward your center line, the linea alba.

To feel this, put your palms on your ribs. If you arch back, belly forward, you might notice your ribs seem to expand and get farther apart. If you stand up neutral, you might sense that your ribs are coming closer together and closer to the center line of your body. Now engage your upper abs and see if you can bring them in a little more, supporting yourself while still standing upright – like putting on a jacket or a cozy sweater and wrapping it around yourself.

---

[9] Inspired by Alicia Pons.

Like a corset of your own making

What if you had the support of a corset, a pair of Spanx®, or a cinched swimsuit – but of your own musculature? A corset of your own making? Engage your abs, your core to support you. Breathe, contract gently, breathe, contract gently. How can you give yourself that feeling of reassurance and support using your own muscles?

Media naranjas – like end caps

Imagine your torso as an orange, split into two halves *(dos media-naranjas)* and then pulled apart to allow room for your organs in between. One half of the sphere is your pelvis and lower abs and the other is your ribcage and shoulder blades. What if we imagine these two half-oranges serving as "end caps" for the structure of our torso, supporting our core on both ends. Engage the low abs and draw up from the pelvic floor at the lower end, and the upper back and upper abs at the other end to stabilize your torso, to contain yourself.

How do your arms feel when you do this? What about your legs? Do they feel free?

Belly breaths

Our diaphragm contracts and pulls downward so that the balloons that are our lungs can inflate. This pushes all those "squishy bits," as Candy Conino likes to call our organs, down and expands our belly. Then the diaphragm releases and parachutes up as the air is expelled from our lungs and our squishy bits have space to come back in and up, so our belly comes in, too.

Place your hands on your belly to feel it expand as you inhale. Can you inhale into your hands? What if you put your hands on your sides – can you inhale into your hands? Hands on your middle back – how would you inhale into your hands there?[10]

As we're working on muscles and support, remember to let them also relax, allowing for those belly breaths. What if you move with awareness of your diaphragm, letting this life-critical, automatic movement "carry" or "lift" you as you go?

---

[10] Inhaling into different parts of the torso was inspired by Ed Mills and Candy Conino.

Rib "basket"

I connected with some lovely folks in Australia during all the pandemic Zoom-ing and learned that what we in the U.S. call the "rib cage", they call a "rib basket". How cool is that? What if we envision our ribs as forming a basket? Perhaps it's a hot air balloon basket. Perhaps we even have a hot air balloon hooked to and lifting our rib basket. Would we float away? How can you move in a way that feels like your rib basket is floating about, hovering gently above the countryside, the hot air balloon casting a small shadow across the tapestry of fields and trees?

Twist

Twist your middle, like a cinnamon twist. We often focus on our movement forward and back, but our spine also can rotate and twist. Great seated or standing. First lengthen – head to heels if standing, or head to tail bone if sitting. Then gently turn your chest and shoulders. If you have space, you might even stretch your arms out to either side. Careful not to collapse your spine as you go. If your twist is small, that's fine. Start where you're at and be gentle with yourself, a little massage for your insides.

Arms like branches

What are your arms doing? Are they sad and wilting, like a plant that hasn't been watered enough – or soggy and limp, like a plant that has been watered too much? What if your arms were like branches, stretching their leaves out to get a glimpse of the sun? What if your arms were like branches, held with poise and purpose?

Welcoming

What if you held your arms open,
palms facing upward,[11]
relaxed?
Welcoming,
ready to receive
all the good stuff
the universe has to offer you.

---

[11] Inspired by Rori Raye.

Thumbs up: no zombies here...

Are you holding your hands like a zombie or the "Thriller"[12] walk? Point one thumb in and down. What happens to your shoulder? Point both thumbs down. What happens to your upper back and chest? Now what if you point your thumbs up? If you're walking, point your thumbs forward and up, like a sprinter pumping their arms. On a leisurely stroll, try pointing those thumbs forward when at your sides and up when swinging in front of your body.

---

[12] The dance in Michael Jackson's "Thriller" video.

Wolverine claws

Are you clenching your fingers? Squeezing your hands tight? Can you make them feel wide, expansive, fingers long and wide, like Wolverine from X-Men?

We often have our toes clenched, too. Stretch them out wide, like webbed duck feet.

And another bowl

If your ribcage can be a bowl, what if your pelvis was also a bowl? Your hips will shift as you walk but what if your overall intention was to keep this bowl facing upright, pelvis level, like a bucket collecting raindrops?

Two bowls

If we have two bowls – rib cage and pelvis – and our body's designed with the intention to maintain balance, then what one bowl does will likely impact the other. If your upper bowl (ribs) is tilted down in front, perhaps your pelvis bowl is also tilted? Is it coming up in the front? Or are they closer to each other in the back?

Bring your sternum and pubic bone closer together (the front of the two bowls closer together). Bring the back of the two bowls closer together (arch the back). Where is a happy medium?

Happy butt, sad butt

"Where is your tailbone?" Alicia Pons will ask in her tango classes. "Is your butt happy, sad, or a little too happy?" Everybody laughs.

Where is your butt? Is it tucked under, pelvis up in front and down in back? Or is your tailbone pointed way out behind you, pelvis tilted down in front, up in the back? How about somewhere in between, a neutral position where your pelvis is about level – a happy but not toooooo happy butt?

Belt buckle

If you had a belt buckle, where would it be
pointing? Is it pointing down toward the
ground? Is it pointing up toward the clouds?
How can you shift which direction your belt
buckle is pointing? What if your belt buckle
pointed straight ahead, like a beacon for where
you are facing, for where you are going?

Sashay

Tight hips can cause all kinds of challenges for our posture. Hips can move side to side, forward and back, up and down. You can make circles with your hips – one side or the whole pelvis.

As you walk, let your hips move. It doesn't have to be a big sashay; simply allow them to absorb the weight shift. Let the impact against the ground travel through your foot, ankle, knee, and hips. It's not how much they move but that they shift as we transfer weight from one leg to the other that is important.

Shake that booty!

Feeling tight in your hips? Shake that booty!
Wiggle your hips. Take a break from whatever
you're doing and shake a little somethin'!
Your body will thank you.

Lots of foot love

We need foot flexibility and strength to adapt to different surfaces and circumstances and set us up for success up the body, too. So give your feet lots of foot love – foot massages, roller balls, calf love, ankle and toe love, too. How we place and use our feet affects our body all the way up… and vice versa. Show your feet some love and attention, some TLC.

Ankle mobility

Your ankle mobility impacts how you stand and walk. Keeping your ankles flexible and strong is super important. Pick up one leg or just lift your foot slightly off the floor and gently turn it, making a circle in one direction, then the other direction. Then switch feet. Heel raises, toe raises will also help. Pointing your toes down like pushing a gas pedal and then up. And of course, most larger foot movements involve the ankle, too. So keep movin'!

Feet were made for... picking things up?

Try to pick things up with your feet. What shall you pick up today? Pick an object (actual or imaginary) and move it from here to there and back again. Or perhaps put it down and then pick up another object. Perhaps you want to knead the floor with your feet, like a cat. You might notice a difference between the agility of one foot and the other.

These movements are great for the front or ball of the foot – the toes, the metatarsals – yet we don't often do them in our daily lives.

Wiggle those toes

Wiggle your toes. If you can put your feet in some grass, do! Enjoy the feeling of the grass tickling your toes. Explore different textures. Perhaps sand or a fluffy rug. Or do this in your fun socks – life is too short for boring socks, after all. Or even if you must – simply *must* – keep your shoes on, wiggle your toes within your shoes. No-one needs to know…

Big toe vs. little toes

Lift your big toe, leaving all your little toes on the ground.

Lift your little toes, leaving your big toe on the ground.[13]

Coordinating this was a challenge for me at first. If it is for you, too, stick with it. Even a small movement counts. It will get easier as your muscles and toes get stronger and more acquainted with the possibilities.

---

[13] Inspired by Pilates teacher Char Powell.

IT'S ALL CONNECTED

The big picture

Mr. Potato Head

When we look at each element of the puzzle and focus on it separately – the hips, feet, shoulders, ankles, toes, head, and so on – we can start to feel disconnected and discombobulated, like the pieces of a Mr. Potato Head toy. We can get confused in the details... Sometimes we need to zoom out for a wider glance, a full-body perspective.

It's all connected, of course

Posture problems are rarely about just one piece of the puzzle.

You can lengthen your neck, for example, from the middle or upper back, start lower and work all the way up. Is your "bowl" tilted? Where are your shoulders? This awareness and small adjustments can make it so much easier to lengthen your neck. Rounded upper back? What is your pelvis doing? Pain in your feet? How are your hips aligned? Are your ribs "stuck" and stiff? The whole system is connected.

Oftentimes by shifting one piece of the puzzle, there are ripple effects up and down the whole structure. Not sure where to start? Try out small changes for size and see how they feel in your body. If something hurts, back off. Let your body be your guide.

Forest vs. trees

It can feel so amazing to get lost in the details, each leaf, each pine needle, each branch... to dive deep into each issue, each nook and cranny, each secret hiding spot. Yet panning out for a wider glance can help orient us, lest we miss the dance of the trees swaying in the wind, the orchestra around us while lost in one pine needle, lest we miss the forest for the trees.

Make room for yourself

Mariana Dragone says our hips stick out and head moves forward because we don't make room for them in the vertical alignment of our body. When we don't lengthen our spines, that's when things get pushed out of the way and are left to find space for themselves. And if we don't make enough room for our boney bits, imagine what's happening to our squishy bits![14]

If instead I stretch my heels toward the floor and the top of my head toward the ceiling, lengthening my spinal column from top to bottom (from my tailbone to the top of my head), all of a sudden, my hips and neck have space to arrange themselves comfortably. When I lengthen my spine and make room for all of me – including all my squishy bits, all the parts of me have space to align.

Try it. Even if you're sitting, you can stretch just your spine. You'll notice right away that your posture improves.[15]

---

[14] I just love Candy Conino's expressions "boney bits" and "squishy bits".

[15] Adapted from Condrea, *When 1+1=1*, pg 43.

Los melones se acomodan solos…

We can get all consumed with placing each melon just so, but *al poner el carrito en marcha, los melones se acomodan solos* – once you get the cart moving, the melons arrange themselves. This saying reminds me of an email chain I received about the golf balls, sand, and coffee in a jar analogy. If you put the sand in first, there isn't room for the golf balls. But if you start with getting the big things in order, there'll be space to fit in the small stuff, too.[16]

---

[16] Adapted from Condrea, *When 1+1=1*, pg 44.

Finding balance

Rounded back? That probably means tight chest muscles and elongated back muscles. Strengthen and shorten the back muscles, stretch, release, and lengthen the chest muscles.

Pelvis tucked under? Perhaps your glutes could use some activation – and the gluteus maximus is the biggest muscle in the whole entire body.

The clue is often in the opposite side of the body. That's where we find balance.

Carry weight using your base

Imagine you're holding heavy kettlebells for resistance training. Using the floor beneath your feet to support yourself all the way up to your shoulders, let your arms relax at your sides. Rather than carrying the kettle-bells by squeezing hard with your hands, engaging intensely in your upper arms, or lifting your shoulders, carry the weight using your base against the floor.

Can you "catch"?

Most of us are pretty good at giving. Receiving is another story. When you feel energy coming your way, do you let it penetrate you, enter your belly, your gut? Are you able to "catch" and receive the energy all the way through to your back, with your whole self, without looking for the exits?

Many of us live our lives out in front of ourselves. I remember dancing at Milonga Barajando in Buenos Aires and choosing something new, a slight shift toward the center of my feet. Tango often emphasizes a forward posture, weight in the balls of the feet. And as good students often do, it is easy to overdo it. With this subtle shift, I could feel the energy into my back, like I was receiving the whole movement – all of it. I could feel it steep inside me for a moment and then I'd choose my response from there. You are strong. You are strong on the inside,[17] you can handle receiving with your whole self. Open, vulnerable, empowered.

---

[17] "Strong on the inside," inspired by Rori Raye.

Like a plant

A plant tells you when it's happy and thriving – or when it feels thirsty, needs light, a little more space. Nurture your body like you would a precious flower in your care.

THE BASE, THE SOURCE

The floor is our friend

The base

Of course, as with any structure, we must consider the base: How are you using your feet? Are you using all the parts of your feet?

If you are sitting, where are you in relation to your sit bones? Find your "own personal"[18] sit bones: right above the crease between the back of your thigh and butt, feel for a pokey bone, one on each side. What if you sit on those and roll back a bit, then roll forward a bit? Then balance right on those pokey sit bones. Which of these three options feels the most solid? In which of these three options does it feel the easiest to lift your chest and head, to be alert and ready?

Do you need to adjust to feel more stable? How can you to take full advantage of the base your body is standing or sitting on right now?

---

[18] "Find your own personal" X, Candy Conino would instruct us anatomy students. The bones of the pelvis (sit bones (ischial tuberosities), ramus of the ischium, and inferior ramus of the pubis), she explained, form an open triangle or V-shape that feels quite stable to rest the upper body on – the slightly forward position mentioned above.

Connect with the floor

Feel the floor under your feet, under each step. How do different surfaces feel? How do you adapt to stepping on concrete, tile, or wood? On uneven surfaces? How do you adapt to going uphill, going downhill? How do your feet, ankles, knees and hips adjust to keep your body upright?

Barefoot

Barefoot, feel the ground, feel the floor under different parts of your feet – the front, the back, the inner edges, outer edges. Receive the support of the ground.

Feel vs. see your feet

Feel your feet. Trust in the connection with the ground – and keep your head up. Trust that whatever comes your way, you and your feet can handle it. Do you need to see them to know they are there, planted solidly on the ground? Feel them.

The floor is our friend

"The floor is our friend," I would tell my walking students. It sounds a little funny – I'd get some giggles – but the floor does support us, and if we let it, it can be our friend. As children, we would crawl and play and bounce on the floor, but as adults we can tend to grow top-heavy, cerebral (all in our heads), and disconnected from the visceral feeling of the relationship with our dear, steady old friend, the floor.

Coins underfoot[19]

Imagine you have coins the size of quarters under your bare feet – one quarter under each of the four corners of each foot: two coins under the ball of the foot, two under the heel. Four coins under each foot makes eight coins total.

Press your feet gently on each quarter, like a little massage, getting reacquainted with the different parts of your feet. Press against one quarter to shift your weight to another quarter. Generate movement in your body by pressing the coin(s). Press the coins to lift your crown.

---

[19] Inspired by Mariana Dragone.

Place weight with emphasis on each toe

Stand or sit. Gently bring your weight forward, shifting weight into one toe, then release, then forward again with weight centered over another toe, release. Work your way from big toe(s) to little toe(s), one toe at a time. Where do you want your weight at this moment? You have the power to choose.[20] From one moment to the next, you have the power to reinvent your connection with your feet.

How you position your upper body can impact where you carry your weight in your lower body and feet, and how you position your feet and the weight in your feet can impact your chest and shoulders, even how you hold your head.[21]

If you feel pain or tightness in the knees, hips, or all the way up, what if you shift where you're putting weight in your foot? Can you find a position that feels good?

---

[20] Inspired by Candy Conino.
[21] Inspired by Ed Mills.

Are you centered?

How is your body weight distributed in your feet? More on one foot than the other? Or if you're sitting, is your weight more on one sit bone than the other?

Shift side to side, feeling your weight to each extreme, to the ends of each side. Then gently find the middle, where your weight is evenly distributed on both sides of your body – both feet or both sit bones. Shoulders and ribcage centered over pelvis centered over feet.

Roots in the ground

Imagine you're growing roots deep into the ground from the soles of your feet. Feel that rooted, grounded connection, like a steady tree. Use it to help you feel solid, stable.

Sea legs

The first time I tried stand-up paddle boarding, I couldn't hold my balance at all. At all. I'd get up and *plop!* In the water I'd go. Enough. I remember deciding that I'd let my lower body (from the waist down – hips, knees, ankles, feet) do a dance to keep my upper body floating. I'd let my lower half adapt to the many intricate changes, the dance of the waves and the constantly shifting surface of the board on the water. I wouldn't try to resist it; I'd go with it. I'd keep my upper body aligned on top and let my lower body do this little dance. And voilà!

DOWN & UP

Where are you going?

If you're walking, you're likely going forward – but are you going forward and up or forward and down? Will you get there faster if you lean forward and down? Probably not.

If you're walking around a corner, notice the position of your upper body. Are you turning right and up or right and down? Left and up or left and down? Which feels more solid in your body?

Like a cat, ready to pounce – or a football player, ready for the snap. Forward and up. Where is your intention?

Superman

"Up, up and away!" like you're Superman or Superwoman and someone's pulling on your cape or your coattails and you're getting ready to take off anyway. Resist the downward pull by pushing the ground.

You're unstoppable.

Trees dance

The branches of a tree are mirrored underground by the roots – and the roots are mirrored by the branches. The branches stretch up and out, roots stretch down and out. Trees seem solid and steady, even rigid. Perhaps we don't think of trees as really moving much. I mean, they don't get up and walk down the street.

But if you watch them on a windy day, their branches dance and sway, the leaves rustle like a symphony. As Autumn comes closer, my friend Christian pointed out one late August day, the leaves start to dry and the sound changes to a drier, sharper, almost a crinkling sound. Trust that your roots, stretching deep into the ground will hold you steady as you let your branches and leaves dance in the wind.

Gravity and the ground beneath our feet

We exist between gravity – or the "fabric of space time curved by the mass of the planet," explains astronomy enthusiast James – and the ground beneath our feet. The pull toward the center of the Earth keeps us from floating away and gives us the resistance against which to maintain the strength and integrity of all our pieces.

Candy Conino pointed out that astronauts have been found to experience adverse effects to blood flow and decreased bone mass, as well as heart and brain function, from prolonged periods in the weightless environment of space. According to the Canadian Space Agency, "on Earth, gravity applies a constant mechanical load to the skeletal system."

The surface beneath us, on the other hand, keeps us from sinking into the molten center of the planet. Using the ground, we can withstand the force of gravity. In fact, our whole standing and sitting life – our whole physical existence – is spent holding ourselves and the integrity of our body structure together in the face of this force. Use it to your advantage.

Because gravity...

If a tree falls in the forest and no-one is around to hear it, does it make a sound? If gravity didn't put pressure on us, would it matter that we stretch and stand tall – to our tallest and fullest potential?

Push down to go up – press against the floor to grow tall.

Handstand prep

When I worked with kids at Seattle Gymnastics Academy prepping them for handstands, we needed to make sure that their arms were ready to hold their body weight, so they wouldn't end up on their heads. Before having them go upside down and fully commit to standing on their hands, we'd often have the class line up, arms extended upward past their ears, palms open flat, facing the ceiling. We'd come push down on their hands. This required them to engage their whole body, from the floor under their feet all the way up through their arms and hands.

Imagine you're prepping for a handstand. Go ahead and stretch your arms up over your head, palms ready to receive a little pressure. Use the ground to help resist this pressure. Then release your arms by your sides, keeping the length in the rest of your body.

Resistance training

Imagine you have a hand pressing down gently on the top of your head. Push the floor to grow taller all the way from the soles of your feet to the top of your head.

Book on head balance

The classic walk with a book on your head. Or sit with a book on your head. And if you don't want to stand out in the crowd or don't have a book handy (hardcover books work best for this), use an imaginary book or object and pretend you are balancing it on your head as you stand, walk, or sit.

Carry water

Imagine you have two cups of water in your
hands, two cups of water balancing on your
shoulders, a jug of water on your head, or
all of the above. You choose. Let your hips,
knees, ankles absorb the shock of each step
as your upper body moves steadily, as if you
were carrying water and didn't want to spill
it. How would you need to stand and move
in order to do that?

Uplifting

I ask my walking students to help lift me up
– or "uplift" me. We "uplift" each other,
pressing down against the ground to lift up.
For many who have been leaning downward
to support themselves on canes and walkers,
this is a big shift in energy. Are you uplifting
yourself – and those around you?

Melt like candlewax

When the muscles in our upper back, chest, and neck are holding tension, we can start to feel top-heavy. When I notice this in my body, I imagine the energy and tension melting, like candlewax. Just let it melt downward toward the middle of my back, where it dissipates. I feel so much lighter right away.

Stretch up and then down

Fill in your chest and upper body like a helium balloon. Stay lifted as you let your pelvis, hips and legs grow heavy and gently ease toward the ground. When I explain this concept to a class, I might even gather my hands close in front of my chest as I breathe in, and then demonstrate a release and gentle opening with my arms as I breathe out and let my lower body settle and ground. Lifted and grounded at the same time, juxtaposing these different, yet complementary sensations.

A floating sensation

"One of the first things I noticed when watching a room full of people dancing tango was that, even though all kinds of fancy things were happening below the waist, they looked like they were floating."[22] It was as if the movements of their lower bodies were dissociated from their upper bodies. While their hips, knees, ankles, and feet absorbed the transfer of weight, their upper bodies seemed to glide effortlessly across the dance floor.

---

[22] Condrea, *When 1+1=1*, 23.

Jumping

I participated in a workshop where we had to jump throughout the day. Between sessions and taking notes and even during the activities, we were jumping. The first day, I felt tired. My shoulders drooped by the end. I could feel the effort of using muscles I hadn't used in forever. The second day felt a little easier and by the fourth day, I felt energized and stronger, like, "I can do this!" Build some jumping, arms up and everything, into your daily routine. Start with say 10-15 a day. In a few days, I bet you'll feel a difference. Ed Mills says that jumping is a great way to reorganize and reorient the body to the sensation of up and down. If you're concerned about joint pain or other health issues, perhaps start with little bounces, gently bending your knees or lifting your heels a bit. Keep your feet or the balls of your feet in contact with the floor, bouncing gently. If this is still too much or if you feel apprehensive, check with your medical provider. It's totally fine to skip this one, too.

EXPAND

Whole wide universe hug

Stretch your arms out wide like a capital "T", like you're showing "I love you *this* much!", like you're so happy you can't contain it.

On top of the mountain

Make yourself into a big "X", stretching far and wide, up and out, like you're standing on top of the mountain, taking it all in.

Take up space

Expand, take up space. Hands on hips.
Expand, breathe into your back.
Expand, yell if you need to. Roar.
Let it all out.

Like fire

dance
stretch, contract
hither, thither
bright
powerful
energy
air and heat
dance, like fire

"Space" in the joints

Create space in the joints. Nothing static, stiff, stuck. Imagine there is fluidity and space between your bones. Do you feel compression in your body? Where can you find and create more spaciousness within yourself? If you find yourself feeling stiff, shake your arms and legs out, stretch big, do a little twist, breathe. No "locking" – always ready to move, dance about the day.

As tall as you can

Stretch as tall as you can on one side, as tall as you can on the other. Reach your arm up, up, up as far as you possibly can... Then the other. Wiggle your hand if you feel inspired. Doesn't it feel good?

Unfurl yourself

Fill in, up and then open. Bring the energy up through your body – a gentle unfolding, expanding, a lifting wave of the arm inspiring the orchestra that is your magnificent body. Sometimes in class, I just motion with my arm like a dancing airport traffic marshaller, and my students straighten up. A visual cue internalized. Subtle. Let it travel up your body, a ripple from your pelvis to your chest, unfurling like a scarf lifted by the wind.

One day, my student Shawn got us all going with his Irish jig. He was working hard and focused on his fancy footwork. Knowing that he likes to say his full name, I asked him, "Who's doin' a Irish jig?"

"I am," he said quietly, still focused on his feet, downward.

"And who's 'I am?'" hand on my hip I asked again, egging him on.

As he started to answer, I motioned a lifting wave in front of my chest. "Shawn Michael Crowley!" he said, standing tall and proud.

Handfuls of cotton candy clouds

Stretch up – maybe even up on your tippy toes – like you're grabbing handfuls of cotton candy clouds from the sky. How often do we as adult humans stretch our arms up?

Center of gravity – a weighted doll

Where is your center of gravity? You can shift your center of gravity depending on how you position your body. You can be more top-heavy, shifting it higher into your chest and shoulders, or more bottom-heavy, shifting it lower into your stomach and pelvis. What feels more steady? What feels like you can stand and walk with ease? Imagine a weighted doll that you push and it sways back and forth and all around, but never topples – grounded, solid, bottom-heavy.

Do the Wave

Reach your arms up as if mimicking a wave with your entire body, all the way up through your fingertips. From standing, arms relaxed at your sides, roll up one vertebra at a time until you end up with your arms reaching up to the sky, like the human wave passed from one section of seats to another, goin' round the baseball stadium.

LET'S TAKE A WALK

Walk

Walking is good for us. It's great for our circulation, gets our blood pumping. Walking helps us maintain mobility, keeps our joints lubricated. Especially executed with good posture, walking keeps us agile and strong. Walking is good for heart, mind, body and soul.

A full-body movement

Walking is a movement that uses all planes. When we walk, we twist, move forward and backward, we stretch across the diagonals of our body. We make cross-body or contralateral connections, up and down connections. Allow it all to happen. Let it all flow.

Look down the road

When you're driving, look down the road. If you look at the hood or "nose" of your car, it'll be harder to drive steadily. You might not see all you need to see for a smooth, safe ride. Look way down the road, using a wide scan and peripheral vision.

So it is with posture, too. Scan wide, breathe, be here and see way down the road ahead of you.

Sternum

Lead from your sternum, dance teachers will say. What if you walk with your sternum – bring it with you. Pay special attention to your sternum. Notice it shifting gently as you walk.[23] Notice it dancing as you step, pointing sightly one way, then the other. Feel the floor-to-sternum connection as your foot lands.

---

[23] Inspired by Ed Mills.

Frankenstein walk

If we're not careful, we can start moving as a block, one whole side at a time, homolaterally like Frankenstein. Instead, let your body gently twist so that the opposite knee and arm come forward at the same time. Revitalize the twist in your body.

The Diagonals

Let your body lengthen along the diagonals as you walk. As you push off of one foot, feel the stretch into the opposite upper "corner" of your body, almost like a long piece of taffy or a rubber band, stretching.

Receive weight with middle back

Feel each step and each movement in your middle back, the space between your shoulder blades. Receive the weight in your feet and up through into each side of the middle of your back as you walk.

Stiff shoulders? Lead with middle back

Sometimes our shoulders stop participating. Perhaps they feel a bit forgotten. Shall we invite them back to the party? Let's include them. Let's let them know we need them, that we love and appreciate them. Walk from the shoulders, focusing on, initiating movement from the center of the back. Lead from the middle of your back, by shifting the shoulders and the back of your ribs, one slightly forward, the other slightly back and switching back and forth. Let your legs follow the motion of your shoulder blades, upper back and the back of your ribs. And your shoulders are back in action!

Let your arms swing

Go for a walk without anything in your hands, free. Let your arms swing, feel the gentle twist of your upper body as you go. Or seated, take a little time to swing one arm forward and the other back, then switch. Keep swinging your arms, alternating.

Lead with your cape

Expand your cape, fling it out behind you. Walk with grandness, creating the storm,[24] encompassing all, leading from your cape, including your whole self, all that your heart desires.

You are the storm.

---

[24] I envision Storm from the X-Men. I envision creating whatever it is my heart desires: passion, creativity, gratitude, joy, strength, presence, "good trouble". What does your heart desire?

Hips are the powerhouse

Hips are the powerhouse, the transition point between the upper body and the lower body, the transition between two legs and one torso. Anchor into the hips as the center of power. Feel the energy move through them as you transition through each phase of a step.

Forward and back

We live so much of our life focused forward, in front of us. Walking is a movement in which if you freeze a person mid-step so you can look at them from the side and drop a line down the middle, you should see part of their body in front of that midline and part of their body behind it. It's almost as if they're stretching themselves in two directions, both forward and backward. When you walk, notice what parts of you go forward, what parts of you go backward, and when.

Do you hear that?

Listen to your feet as they meet the ground with each step. What does it sound like? Do they shuffle along, the front part sort of sliding or grinding into the pavement? Does your heel drag a bit, scraping? Do they land heavy, like a tired elephant? Perhaps you hear a soft caressing or a pitter-patter as you step? Can you make a different sound with your feet? What shifts in your upper body change how your feet come in contact with the ground? Which sound-and-posture combination feels best in your body right now?

Walk like you are a thick, syrupy molasses, or taffy, water, melted chocolate… you choose. Use the ground under your feet to move yourself forward through whichever substance you choose to walk through or be.

Walk like you're in charge, the boss. You are the boss of you. Own each step. There is plenty of space for each of us to be and to thrive.

Walk with density, weight in your feet, aplomb. Step, like you mean it. Upper body lifted, light.

A walk through your body

Travel your awareness throughout your body. Focus on different body parts as you walk, stand, sit. Go on a journey head to toe through your body – or toes to head, or shift your focus bouncing from one place to another in no particular order, as you feel inspired. Listen to your body. Where are my shoulders? Hips? How does my neck feel? Do I feel pain or tension anywhere? How do I feel in my body right now? Allow yourself to just be with yourself – an intimate journey of being in your body. Build awareness.

AWARENESS

Move with joy

Breathe

Are you breathing? I was going about my garden one day, clipping this, weeding that, tending my little green world, and I told myself, Today, I'm just going to pay attention to whether I'm breathing or holding my breath. And if I notice I'm holding my breath? Simple: breathe. Go about your day and just notice your breathing. If you catch yourself holding your breath or breathing shallow, just pause, acknowledge it, and breathe.

Symmetry

Notice any asymmetrical position you tend to hold. For example, I often contort my body when I write. I'm right-handed, so I favor one side over the other. I twist my head and upper body, angle the page. Perhaps you love a sport or activity that is asymmetrical, like tango, golf, bowling... What can you do to balance this? Perhaps from time to time, twist the other way, or realign your shoulders, or stand and do something full-body or completely different as a break and to "reset".

Are your shoulders level?

If you had two cups of water, one resting on each shoulder, would they be spilling to one side or the other? What about your hips? Are you holding one side of your body shorter than the other?

Body scan

Scan your body. Where do you feel tension? "Ahhh… I feel tension in X." Rori Raye says rather than fight the tension or get upset or frustrated about it, say to that part of yourself, "I love the part of myself that wants to get things right, or that feels overwhelmed, or that's just trying to hold it all together." Place your hand on the spot or simply feel into it without even touching it. Breathe into it. Let it go. Let the muscles release, let the tension melt away.

In motion and rest

Our bodies need
both

to
rest,
replenish,
re-energize,
relax

and

to
engage,
be active,
fire those muscle spindles.

Move with joy.

(What's the alternative?)

Dance party

In your seat, at your desk, in the kitchen, walking down the street. Shift your weight side to side from one foot to the other or one butt cheek to another and have yourself a little "dance party", as my student Ellie likes to call it. Do a little jig, as Shawn says. Your body will thank you!

Put on some music that moves you or dance to the music in your soul...

Move your body

We want our bodies to do a lot for us, don't we? We need to give our body what it needs:

Movement. We're not designed to sit for hours on end.

Play. Movement and living in your body should feel good – for you and all your cells. When you move, you bring vital nutrients to your whole system.

Rest. If we want to move well, stand well, sit well, we need our muscles to help make that happen, so, in turn, they also need to rest well.

Move well.
Eat well.
Rest well.
Be well.

Living is an active, participatory pursuit.

Move like you mean it

Are you engaging your muscles while you sit, stand, talk to a friend? Not that you need to always be getting ready to lift heavy weights – not that kind of engaged, but it does take muscles to hold ourselves up. Are you engaging them gently, enough to stand, sit, walk, move, dance effectively? Are you moving like you mean it?

Rest like you mean it

Lie down, lounge, relax, sit back in your chair. Let something – the ground, a mattress, a cushy couch – support you. If you need to rest or desire to rest, do rest.

Collapsing dolls

You know the dolls where you press a button and they stand tall, but when you let go of the button, they sort of crumble? We don't want to be those dolls except when we purposely take much-needed rest. But if you're standing up, sitting up, or walking, engage your muscles to counter any collapsing feeling, especially from your hips and up. You've got this.

No Eeyore[25] in your posture...

Have you that sinking feeling? Do you catch yourself leaning or "sinking" into objects – the counter, your chair, armrest – or people? Kind of feels energetically miserable and draining, doesn't it? When you're standing or sitting, see if you can engage your muscles to hold you. Try to be "on" or "off" – not halfway slumping, neither here nor there, neither active and engaged nor resting. Slow and deliberate or slow and soft are a different feeling than slow and dragging. If you're feeling like Eeyore, do something to soothe your soul, self-care, ask for help, give yourself what you need... and then go and get what you want.

---

[25] Referring to Winnie-the-Pooh's friend, who is generally characterized as being sad and droopy.

Use it or lose it

We are efficient machines. Your muscles came here to work! When muscles are being used, it's clear that the movement is needed, so those muscles are nurtured. Joints get fluid and lubrication as we use them, too. But muscles that are neglected shrivel. If you don't use them, your brain and nervous system assumes you don't need them. Over time, muscles that aren't engaged get weaker, smaller, and atrophy. And if you don't need them, they must be pruned and gotten rid of, the brain thinks. It's spring cleaning.

Like a garden, what you nurture grows. Use it or lose it.

Rest on purpose, move with purpose

Rest is so important, and I really encourage my walking students to pay attention to their energy level and advocate for themselves when they need a break. For those who need a lot of support, this is crucial – they need to make it back to their chair safely, for all our sake. Yet, when they're up, they must work. Leaning and pushing on me like they would a walker or cane is not sustainable for me or a caregiver or volunteer and not ideal long-term for the student either. When they stand, they stand tall. Ask yourself: Am I slumping or slouching because I'm tired and need to rest? Then take a rest – even a short rest can help. Or do I have the energy to stand stronger, taller, more solidly on my feet? If it's the second one, then hop to! Let's do this!

Take breaks –

rest breaks and movement breaks.

And stretch breaks. Mmm…

Check in

Ask yourself, how would my X (a body part – shoulder, for example) like to move?[26] Be gentle. Perhaps little circles, getting gradually bigger. Perhaps a back-and-forth linear movement, like you're scratching something out on paper. Perhaps you doodle, move and pause. What does your (shoulder) want? What does your shoulder need?

---

[26] Inspired by Erica Eickhoff & Rori Raye.

Taking someone else's space[27]

When it comes to our own individual space, we have all probably had the sensation that things might be easier if we took up less space. The fact is that many, many of us do take up too much space, and it has nothing to do with that extra slice of pizza you ate or the fact that some of us have larger hips than others. Many of us take up more space than our natural body composition would require due to our poor posture.

If you've ever taken a dance class, you've probably heard a teacher say, Don't look at your feet! Keep your head up! And the class would obediently lift their heads for just a moment before sinking into the same inclination to look at what marvelous things were happening with their feet. But one day, I heard Olga Besio say, "If you look down, you're taking someone else's space." Wow! A totally different perspective: If my head is not aligned on top of my spine and I'm hunched over, I am taking someone else's space.

---

[27] Adapted from Condrea, *When 1+1=1*, 43.

Own your space

On a crowded dance floor or a crowded sidewalk – just as on an empty stage – even energetically, own your space. We are each worthy and deserving of the space we occupy on this planet and in our communities, our families, and daily lives. **And those around us are impacted by the manner in which we carry ourselves.** When we are clear in our space, it helps others get their bearings, too. For yourself and for those around you, own your space.

SELF-CONNECTION

Posture, inside-out

Posture is self-care 101. Put on your oxygen mask.

Our inner world and outward physical expression are intimately intertwined

How you feel on the inside will express itself on the outside. My mom would say when trying to convince me as a little girl that I needed to wear a coat, "If you don't feel good, you won't look good. And if you feel good" – warm enough – "you'll look good, too."

If we don't feel congruent, it's hard to "fake it". Do the inner work – work on the self-connection and it will reflect on the outside, too.

Am I ok?!

"Are you ok?" El Chino Perico would check in after a song.

"Yes, very!"

"Ok, good."

Ok?! Dancing with the dapper and refined gentleman El Chino, I was floating on a cloud, like a dream.

He is wise. If I am feeling good, he'll have an easier time dancing with me. Just him asking me if I feel good puts my nerves at ease. I can feel my whole self relax.

We can do this for ourselves, too. Check in with yourself. Take good care of yourself. If you are well, everyone around you benefits.

Be present

Between what was and what will be, you are, Rodolfo Dinzel would tell us. Work the middle between the front of you (the future) and the back of you (your past). Stand, move from that place and awareness, embodying the space you occupy.

The posture of fear

Trauma big and small can cause us to feel fearful, which compels us to protect ourselves. People will often adopt a protective stance after a fall or if they feel unsteady on their feet or unsteady in themselves, curled inward toward the fetal position (even slightly). It gives the sensation of protecting the vital organs. In some cases, people still live in response to the trauma even when the incident has passed. Wounds can become ingrained in how we carry ourselves. Emotional scars. Ironically, this posture can produce less steadiness, more problems with balance – and more fear.

What if we could start a gentle, gradual unfolding – slowly opening up, learning to trust our feet again, learning to trust ourselves again?

The Thinker

Is it necessary to be curled inward to focus, like "The Thinker" statue? Does one have to position oneself with a rounded back to contemplate and focus? Can one stretch and focus? Can one hold their space and focus? Be open and present and focused?

Closed off or rejecting?

Arch forward, arch backward. One extreme feels closed off, protective, guarded, not letting anyone or anything in – or even sucking energy, like a vampire. At the other extreme, it's like ice, rejecting, an impenetrable forcefield. Maintaining the flexibility to execute each extreme is great, yet we don't want to live – or stand or sit – in either of these all the time. Find a neutral place in between: brave, grounded, openhearted.

Receive with grace for yourself

Years ago, I saw myself on a video of a presentation I did for the ASU Tango Club in a beautiful art gallery packed with people. I remember feeling nervous, as I always do getting up to speak. Later, watching the video, I noticed my rounded upper back, as if subconsciously I was trying to make myself less obtrusive. I wanted to share my message, my work, yet in the face of all that attention, I saw myself not fully owning the space. It was so clearly reflected in my posture.

When the emotions feel intense, when it feels like too much to bear, challenge yourself to stay open, stand strong, rooted… and trust that if you really need to, you can take care of yourself. If you need to move away from something truly bad for you, you will. But if it's too much good stuff, challenge yourself to receive just a little more at a time, to remain unguarded, allow the energy to flow through you, and come out in beautiful, unexpected ways. Don't try to contain it. Surrender. Receive with grace for yourself.

"No te achiques"

"No te achiques," Chiche said to me while we were dancing swing – "don't make yourself smaller." Chiche noticed I'd shrink, self-conscious. I don't know how to dance swing, I'd said to myself and confessed to him. And the older folks at the milonga moved so smoothly, like their bodies were floating, even in swing! I felt unsteady and unsure.

Yet, the truth is that making yourself smaller does not help you dance swing any better – in fact, it does the opposite. So it is in life, in anything we do. Be open, be humble, keep learning – and stand tall each step of the way. You don't have to be small to be receptive.

Chiche's encouragement gave me confidence in an unconfident space, so I say it to you, as well: *"No te achiques."*

Don't "short-change" us!

"Stand up tall," Debbie and I remind Gus in class.

"Don't short-change us," I say.

"Yeah, we want all 6'1" of you!" Debbie adds.

Gus laughs and stands taller.

Especially if you tend to tower over people around you, stand tall. Do not shrink to get closer, to blend in. Connect – with your full self, each and every inch of you. Stand tall, dance, walk, show up with all of yourself – with your whole self. Bring your whole self to the table.

Love yourself, all the parts of yourself[28]

Even if you see "more" of yourself in the mirror than you'd like – if you notice a little extra here and a little extra there. Or maybe you've just been through some changes in your body. It is all part of you. Standing smaller will not make you less noticeable or any perceived imperfections less visible. Embrace it. Embrace yourself. Do what you need to do to feel healthy, to feel good. And embrace yourself – all the parts of yourself – now and each step of the way.

---

[28] Inspired by Adrienne Everheart, who recommends saying to yourself: "I love myself, all the parts of myself."

Let your light shine

Your playing small serves no-one.[29] Where are you holding back? What part of you is "hiding in plain sight"?[30] Don't dim your light. There's plenty of room under the sun for everyone.[31]

---

[29] Inspired by Marianne Williamson's poem "Our deepest fear".

[30] Inspired by Jamie Kern Lima.

[31] Inspired by my Unchiu Glebus Sainciuc.

Tits up, sis!

No matter what size or shape, if you have breasts, you might be part of the contingent that tries (consciously or subconsciously) to hide them. If this is you, or if this resonates for you in any way, this cue is for you: Tits up, sis![32]

---

[32] "Tits up" is a term used in show biz before going on stage. Its incorporation here was inspired by Jenna Beem who was inspired by The Marvelous Mrs. Maisel.

Worthiness

Relaxing into the space you occupy, presence. A sense of fullness, worthiness, grandness. It is ok for you to be here – in fact, it is important. Touch an object, observe your surroundings, take in the sounds. Trust you are in exactly the right place at exactly the right time.[33] And you are plenty. You are more than enough.

---

[33] Inspired by Helena Hart.

Like setting goals for yourself

Posture is not just about the here and now (short-term goals); it's also about the big picture: Where are you going? How are you setting yourself up now to get there in a way that feels good?

Heart connection

Connect with the world with your heart wide open, expansive. Play an instrument, give a speech, do a dance, stand, walk, run – with your heart wide open. Create a deep heart-to-heart connection with any and everything you do, be, are.

Posture is a dance, so keep "boogie-ing on down the road!" says TangoStride student Shawn Michael Crowley.

Thank You

To all the teachers and coaches – named in this book and not – who have shaped and enriched my teaching and my posture practice.

To all my tango students, for the honor of being a part of your journey. A special shout-out to my TangoStride students, for your trust and courage. You each keep me going on this path. A heart full of gratitude to you!

To my editors Lydia Condrea and Terry Benioff, who really "get" me. I feel so fortunate to be able to share my writing with you and appreciate your thoughtful and meticulous feedback. This book would not have been possible without you! And Iris. Toby surely would've helped, too.

To my study-buddy Erica, my accountability partner Kevin, Monica and William for a room to write in, Jenna and Kaia for your support during the formatting process, and Sami Wunder for the empowered energy inspiration.

To the Seattle tango community for all your support over the years. Special thanks to the TangoHappyHour Crew and the supporters of Hugs that Empower nonprofit for making our TangoStride work possible.

To my friends in Seattle, in Argentina, and everywhere in between, for your support, hugs, and feedback. Special shout-out to my friends who are like family. It takes a village – thank you for being my village.

To my family, near and far, mulțumesc. A special thank you for all your invaluable gifts: Bunicul Constantin "Carol" Condrea, who encouraged me to observe the world around me and write, to Bunica Caty and Bunicul Vlad and my parents Lydia and Arcady Condrea, for their love of movement, to Bunica Raia for modeling awareness, to Aunt Inna-Sabrina for all the laughs and encouragement, to my "big" brother Daniel for taking care of house projects while I wrote, to Tanti Valentina Rusu-Ciobanu and Unchiu Glebus Sainciuc, who encouraged us little ones to draw and paint, and Aunt Genya, who enjoyed the little things and lived with such a big heart. A special shout-out again to my Mom for dealing with my endless requests for feedback and encouraging agency in my art from a very young age, and to my Dad for his courage and determination.

To all the many people I have not mentioned here – for each conversation, each interaction that inspired the creation of this book, thank you! Thank you so very much!